The Healing Power of Fruits

Diet to Beat Disease and Defy Aging

Willow Morgan

TABLE OF CONTENTS

Chapter Three
THE HEALING MAGIC OF FRUITS
A dive into the health benefits of various fruits.
Fruit healing properties and how they can aid in curing diseases.
Real-life success stories and testimonials.

Chapter Four
BALANCED NUTRITION BEYOND FRUITS
Explore a variety of other foods that complement the fruit-based diet.
Discuss the importance of a balanced nutritional intake and how it contributes to overall health.

Chapter Five
FIGHTING THE BATTLE OF THE BULGE:
Weight Management
How a food and fruit diet can aid in weight loss and weight management.
Practical tips and meal plans designed to assist in shedding excess weight.

Chapter Six
DEFYING TIME:
Anti-Aging Secrets
The anti-aging benefits of a fruit and food diet, such as antioxidants and nutrients that combat signs of aging.
Expert advice on maintaining youthful vitality through dietary choices.

Chapter Seven
TARGETING AILMENTS
A Diet for Disease Prevention and Recovery
How a food and fruit diet can help prevent and manage various diseases.
Specific dietary recommendations for common health issues.

Chapter Eight
IMPLEMENTING THE DIET
A step-by-step guide on transitioning to and maintaining a food and fruit diet.
Practical tips, tricks, and strategies for success.

Chapter Twelve
KEY TAKEAWAYS FROM THIS BOOK
Embark on your own journey toward better health using the insights and tools provided in this book.

INTRODUCTION:

Picture this: a woman, burdened with chronic illnesses and the weight of her ailments. She had tried countless medications, doctor visits, and expensive treatments, but nothing seemed to offer lasting relief. She felt trapped and resigned to a life of constant struggle. But her life changed the day she discovered the incredible potential of fruits as medicine.

In the pages that follow, we invite you to embark on a deeply personal voyage of transformation. Through myriads of experiences, coupled with remarkable success stories shared by individuals just like you, we will explore how fruits -- yes, the very sustenance we consume each day -- possesses an astonishing power to heal, rejuvenate, and restore our bodies and minds.

Imagine the awe-inspiring journey of Thomas, an individual burdened by the weight of diabetes and obesity. Conventional treatments offered him little hope, until he decided to embrace a diet rich in fruits and wholesome foods. Witness his gradual shedding of excess weight, his newfound energy and vitality, as his blood sugar levels stabilize and his zest for life reignites. Thomas, like countless others, discovered a beacon of hope in the transformative power of fruits.

Or consider Michelle, who spent years battling both an autoimmune disorder and the often-debilitating symptoms of aging. Her body was a battleground, until she immersed herself in the world of nutrition and holistic healing. Embracing a diet brimming with antioxidant-rich fruits, she experienced a remarkable reversal of her symptoms. Today, Michelle radiates with youthfulness, her spirits lifted, and her once-painful joints now nimble.

These stories are not anomalies; they are shining examples of the stunning potential that lies within the very meals we consume. The fruits we eat possess an incredible ability to empower our bodies, strengthen our immune systems, and control our weight. They offer us a lifeline to defy the burdens of aging and protect ourselves against the onslaught of diseases.

In this captivating book, we will journey through the science, wisdom, and practicality of harnessing the transformative power of fruits. From unraveling the core principles behind nutrition to providing you with tools and strategies to create personalized meal plans, we leave no stone unturned in our quest for lasting health and vitality.

As you turn the pages, you will discover not just the scientific evidence, but also a bountiful chest of personal anecdotes, success stories, and real-life experiences that will resonate with your own journey. These stories will inspire you, ignite your curiosity, and demonstrate the remarkable transformations that are within your reach.

So, dear reader, are you prepared to leave behind the path of uncertainty and embrace an extraordinary journey toward lasting health and vitality? Join me as we unlock the secrets that lie within your plate, creating a life of fulfillment and well-being. The time has come to seize control of your health destiny. Let us embark together on this captivating adventure, where the power to transform awaits you.

Chapter One
NATURE'S PALETTE: UNVEILING THE HEALING POWER OF FRUITS

In a world brimming with possibilities, the answer to a healthier, more vibrant life often lies in the simple and the unassuming. Picture a farmer's market on a bustling morning—the kaleidoscope of colors and the symphony of aromas swirling around you. Welcome to nature's own art gallery, where the canvas is painted with the hues of fruits, and the brushstrokes are strokes of health and vitality.

Each fruit, a jewel in nature's treasure trove, offers not just flavor and nourishment but a myriad of healing wonders. From the fiery red of a ripe strawberry to the calming green of a juicy kiwi, these natural miracles hold the potential to rejuvenate our bodies and uplift our spirits. In this chapter, we'll delve into this vibrant palette and discover how these colorful gifts from nature can revolutionize our well-being.

As we journey through the spectrum of fruits, we'll unlock the secrets of their nutritional prowess. From antioxidants that combat the ravages of time to vitamins that fortify our immune systems, each bite is a step towards a stronger, healthier you. Let's peel back the layers, slice through the myths, and savor the wisdom that nature has bestowed upon us.

Join me in this exciting adventure through the orchards and groves, where we'll feast not just on fruits but on the promise of a better, more invigorated life. The table is set, and the fruits are ripe for the picking—let the colorful odyssey begin!

Chapter Two
THE ESSENCE OF HEALTH

Understanding the Foundation

In our quest for health and vitality, it's vital to understand the very foundation upon which our journey rests. The fruit and food diet isn't just a collection of meals; it's a philosophy, a science, and a lifestyle rolled into one. In this chapter, we'll unravel the essence of this transformative approach to eating.

The Science behind the Diet

Before we dive into the practical aspects, let's grasp the science that underpins the fruit and food diet. At its core, this dietary choice is rooted in the belief that the healing power of nature can be harnessed through fruits. From phytonutrients to fiber, fruits provide us with an array of compounds that nurture our bodies and fend off diseases.

These natural wonders are not merely sustenance; they are medicine in edible form.

The Principles that Guide Us

Now, let's explore the principles that govern this lifestyle. The fruit and food diet places emphasis on fresh, whole foods, steering clear of processed and artificial substances. It embraces the wisdom of mindful eating, encouraging us to savor each bite, connect with the source of our sustenance, and be present in the act of nourishing ourselves.

A Journey toward Healing

This diet is not just about physical health; it's a holistic approach that considers the well-being of mind and spirit too. By consuming fruits in their most natural state, we allow our bodies to heal and rejuvenate. It's a lifestyle that invites us to pause, reflect, and truly savor the essence of life.

The Spectrum of Foods

While fruits take center stage, a food and fruit diet isn't limited to them alone. We also explore the world of vegetables, grains, and legumes—all of which have a role to play in our journey towards wellness. Balancing our nutritional intake is key, and this diet ensures we get a diverse array of nutrients.

A Glimpse into What Lies Ahead

As we venture deeper into this diet, we'll discover its power to heal ailments, fight the battle against aging, and address the issue of excess weight. The journey is rich with flavors, knowledge, and transformation. So, fasten your seatbelt and prepare to embark on a path that promises not just health but a profound connection with the nourishing essence of life itself. The fruit and food diet is not just a choice; it's a commitment to thriving, and our journey has only just begun.

Deciphering the food and fruit diets we need for daily living

Deciphering the right food and fruit diets for daily living involves understanding your nutritional needs, dietary preferences, and overall health goals. Here's a step-by-step approach to guide you:

Assess Your Nutritional Needs:

Consider your age, gender, activity level, and overall health.

Consult a healthcare professional or a registered dietitian for a personalized assessment.

Understand Macronutrients:

Learn about macronutrients: carbohydrates, proteins, and fats, and their importance in your diet.

Balance these macronutrients according to your needs and goals.

Explore Micronutrients:

Familiarize yourself with essential micronutrients like vitamins and minerals and their roles in your body.
Include a variety of fruits and vegetables to ensure you get a broad spectrum of micronutrients.

Consider Dietary Preferences:

Account for dietary restrictions, allergies, or ethical choices (e.g., vegetarian, vegan, gluten-free).
Choose foods and fruits that align with your preferences while meeting your nutritional requirements.

Include a Variety of Fruits:

Incorporate a colorful array of fruits to ensure you benefit from various antioxidants, vitamins, and minerals.

Aim for diversity in fruit types to cover a broad nutritional spectrum.

Portion Control and Moderation:

Practice portion control to avoid overeating and maintain a healthy weight.
Enjoy fruits and other foods in moderation to maintain a balanced diet.
Listen to Your Body:

Pay attention to your body's hunger and fullness cues.
Adjust your diet based on how different foods make you feel and how they impact your energy levels.
Stay Hydrated:

Incorporate plenty of water and hydrating fruits in your daily routine to support overall well-being.
Meal Planning:

Plan your meals ahead, incorporating a mix of fruits, vegetables, whole grains, lean proteins, and healthy fats.

Prepare a shopping list to ensure you have nutritious options readily available.
Regular Exercise:

Integrate regular physical activity into your routine for optimal health and weight management, complementing your dietary choices.

Seek Professional Guidance:

If you have specific health concerns, consult a healthcare professional or a registered dietitian for expert advice and a personalized diet plan.
Adopting a balanced and mindful approach to food and fruit consumption, tailored to your unique needs and preferences, will contribute to a healthier and fulfilling daily life.

Food and fruit diets and its key principles

A food and fruit diet is a dietary approach that emphasizes the consumption of a variety of fresh, whole fruits and vegetables, along with other wholesome foods like whole grains, legumes, nuts, seeds, and lean proteins. The diet minimizes or eliminates processed foods, refined sugars, unhealthy fats, and excessive animal products. Key principles of this diet include:

Whole, Unprocessed Foods:

The diet encourages the consumption of whole, minimally processed foods to retain their natural nutrients and health benefits.
Plant-Centric Approach:

Fruits and vegetables form a significant portion of the diet, providing essential vitamins, minerals, fiber, and antioxidants.

Diverse Nutrition:

A variety of fruits and vegetables are recommended to ensure a broad spectrum of nutrients necessary for overall health and well-being.

Balanced Macronutrients:

The diet aims for a balanced intake of carbohydrates, proteins, and healthy fats from plant-based sources.
Mindful Eating:

Practicing mindful eating, savoring each bite, and listening to the body's hunger and fullness cues are encouraged.

Hydration:

Adequate water intake, often complemented by hydrating fruits, is emphasized for optimal health and vitality.

Customization:

The diet can be customized to individual needs, considering factors like dietary preferences, health conditions, and lifestyle choices.

The Science Behind Healing, Anti-Aging, and Weight Loss:

Healing Properties:

Many fruits and vegetables are rich in vitamins, minerals, antioxidants, and phytonutrients known for their healing properties.
Antioxidants combat harmful free radicals in the body, reducing the risk of chronic diseases and supporting cellular repair and regeneration.

Anti-Aging Benefits:

Antioxidants, vitamins, and minerals found abundantly in fruits and vegetables can help neutralize free radicals that accelerate the aging process.
Certain fruits contain compounds that promote collagen production and maintain skin elasticity, contributing to a youthful appearance.

Aiding Weight Loss:

Fruits and vegetables are typically low in calories and high in fiber, promoting a

feeling of fullness and aiding in weight management.
Fiber slows down digestion, reducing hunger and preventing overeating. Additionally, fiber supports a healthy gut microbiome, which is linked to weight control.
Nutrient Density:

Fruits and vegetables are nutrient-dense, providing a wide array of essential vitamins, minerals, and micronutrients per calorie consumed.
Nutrient-dense foods offer satiety while ensuring the body receives the necessary nutrients for optimal functioning.
By understanding these principles and the scientific basis behind the benefits of a fruit and food diet, individuals can make informed choices to improve their overall health, combat aging, and manage their weight effectively.

Chapter Three
THE HEALING MAGIC OF FRUITS

A dive into the health benefits of various fruits.
Fruits healing properties and how they can aid in curing diseases.
Real-life success stories and testimonials.

Blueberries:

Health Benefits:

Blueberries are packed with antioxidants, particularly anthocyanins, which combat oxidative stress and reduce the risk of chronic diseases.
They support brain health, improve memory, and may reduce the risk of age-related cognitive decline.

Blueberries have anti-inflammatory properties and may help manage blood sugar levels.
Real-Life Success Story:

Mark, a 60-year-old retiree, incorporated blueberries into his daily diet. Over time, he noticed improved mental clarity and felt more energetic. His cholesterol levels also decreased, indicating better heart health.

Avocado:

Health Benefits:

Avocados are rich in healthy monounsaturated fats that support heart health and may help lower bad cholesterol levels.
They are a good source of fiber, aiding in digestion and promoting a feeling of fullness.
Avocados contain vitamins C, E, K, and B-6, contributing to a strong immune system and healthy skin.
Real-Life Success Story:

Sarah struggled with cholesterol issues. By incorporating avocados into her diet, along with a balanced lifestyle, she managed to reduce her LDL cholesterol levels significantly, impressing her doctor during her checkup.

Oranges:

Health Benefits:

Oranges are an excellent source of vitamin C, supporting the immune system, skin health, and wound healing.
They contain fiber and potassium, promoting heart health and regulating blood pressure.
Oranges are rich in antioxidants, helping combat free radicals and reducing the risk of chronic diseases.
Real-Life Success Story:

David, a fitness enthusiast, started consuming oranges daily after workouts. He noticed a boost in his immune system, fewer post-exercise muscle cramps, and increased energy levels, allowing him to intensify his workout routine.

Strawberries:

Health Benefits:

Strawberries are high in vitamin C and antioxidants, supporting the immune system and fighting free radicals.
They contain anthocyanins and ellagic acid, potentially reducing the risk of heart disease and certain cancers.
Strawberries are low in calories and high in fiber, aiding in weight management and digestion.
Real-Life Success Story:

Emily struggled with digestive issues and incorporated strawberries into her daily meals. The fiber content helped regulate her digestion, and she experienced less bloating and discomfort.
These real-life success stories and testimonials demonstrate how integrating these fruits into one's diet can positively

impact health and well-being. It's important to consult a healthcare professional before making significant dietary changes, especially for individuals with existing health conditions.

Bananas:

Health Benefits:

Bananas are a great source of potassium, essential for heart health, maintaining blood pressure, and balancing electrolytes.
They provide a quick energy boost due to their natural sugars, making them an excellent pre-workout snack.
Bananas contain vitamin B6, aiding brain function and the production of neurotransmitters.
Real-Life Success Story:

Michael, a busy professional, struggled with low energy levels during the day. After adding bananas to his daily routine, he felt more energized and experienced fewer midday slumps, enhancing his productivity.

Apples:

Health Benefits:

Apples are rich in fiber, aiding in digestion, promoting a feeling of fullness, and supporting gut health.
They contain antioxidants and phytochemicals that may lower the risk of chronic diseases, including heart disease and diabetes.
Apples may help regulate blood sugar levels and support weight management.
Real-Life Success Story:

Rachel, a diabetes patient, began incorporating apples into her diet. With consistent monitoring and a balanced diet, she observed better blood sugar control and a reduction in her HbA1c levels.

Pineapples:

Health Benefits:

Pineapples are a rich source of vitamin C, aiding the immune system and promoting wound healing.
They contain bromelain, an enzyme that may help with digestion and reduce inflammation.
Pineapples are low in calories and high in water content, making them a hydrating and satisfying snack.
Real-Life Success Story:

Jason struggled with digestive discomfort. After incorporating pineapples into his diet, he noticed reduced bloating and improved digestion, allowing him to feel more comfortable after meals.

Grapes:

Health Benefits:

Grapes are high in antioxidants, including resveratrol, which may have heart-protective effects and reduce the risk of certain cancers. They are a natural source of hydration due to their high water content, aiding in kidney function and detoxification.
Grapes contain vitamins C and K, supporting immune health and bone health, respectively.
Real-Life Success Story:

Lisa, dealing with a family history of heart disease, included grapes as a daily snack. Over time, her cholesterol levels improved, and her cardiologist noted the positive impact on her heart health during check-ups. These success stories and the associated health benefits of various fruits showcase how incorporating a diverse range of fruits into one's diet can lead to improved health outcomes and overall well-being. It's essential to listen to your body's responses and consult a healthcare professional for personalized advice and guidance.

CHAPTER FOUR
BALANCED NUTRITION BEYOND FRUITS
Exploring a variety of other foods that complement the fruit-based diet
The importance of a balanced nutritional intake and how it contributes to overall health

In addition to fruits, a balanced fruit-based diet should include a variety of other foods to ensure a well-rounded and complete nutritional intake. Here's an exploration of these complementary foods and the significance of a balanced nutritional intake for overall health:

1. Vegetables:

Importance: Vegetables are rich in vitamins, minerals, fiber, and antioxidants essential for overall health. They support immune function, digestion, and reduce the risk of chronic diseases.

Inclusion: Include a colorful array of vegetables like leafy greens, carrots, bell peppers, broccoli, and spinach in your meals for optimal nutrition.

2. Whole Grains:

Importance: Whole grains provide complex carbohydrates, fiber, vitamins, and minerals. They promote digestive health, regulate blood sugar levels, and offer sustained energy.

Inclusion: Incorporate whole grains like quinoa, brown rice, whole wheat, oats, and barley in your meals for a balanced diet.

3. Legumes and Pulses:

Importance: Legumes are rich in protein, fiber, iron, and folate. They support muscle growth, provide sustained energy, and aid in digestion and heart health.

Inclusion: Include lentils, chickpeas, black beans, and peas to add plant-based protein to your diet.

4. Nuts and Seeds:

Importance: Nuts and seeds offer healthy fats, protein, vitamins, and minerals. They support brain function, heart health, and help manage weight.

Inclusion: Include almonds, walnuts, chia seeds, flaxseeds, and pumpkin seeds as snacks or toppings to your meals.

5. Lean Proteins:

Importance: Lean proteins like poultry, fish, tofu, and low-fat dairy provide essential amino acids for muscle repair, immune function, and hormone production.

Inclusion: Incorporate lean protein sources to support muscle maintenance and overall body strength.

6. Dairy or Dairy Alternatives:

Importance: Dairy products or fortified dairy alternatives like almond milk or soy milk provide calcium, protein, and essential vitamins for bone health and overall growth.

Inclusion: Consume low-fat or non-fat dairy, or fortified dairy alternatives to meet calcium and protein requirements.

7. Healthy Fats:

Importance: Healthy fats like those found in avocados, olive oil, and fatty fish are essential for heart health, brain function, and hormone balance.

Inclusion: Use these fats in moderation to support overall well-being.

Importance of a Balanced Nutritional Intake:

Overall Health: A balanced diet ensures the body receives a diverse range of nutrients necessary for growth, repair, and optimal function of organs and systems.

Disease Prevention: A well-rounded diet can help prevent or manage chronic diseases like diabetes, heart disease, and certain cancers.

Energy and Vitality: Proper nutrition provides the energy needed for daily activities, enhances mood, and promotes a sense of vitality and well-being.

Immune Support: A variety of nutrients from different food groups strengthen the immune system, helping the body fight off infections and illnesses.

Incorporating a variety of foods into a fruit-based diet is key to achieving a balanced nutritional intake, supporting overall health, and promoting a robust and active lifestyle.

CHAPTER FIVE
FIGHTING THE BATTLE OF THE BULGE
How a fruit and food diet can aid in weight loss and weight management.
Practical tips and meal plans designed to assist in shedding excess weight.

A food and fruit diet can aid in weight loss and weight management due to its emphasis on whole, unprocessed foods, and the inclusion of fruits, which are typically low in calories and high in fiber. Here's how it can be effective:

Low Caloric Density: Fruits and vegetables are low in calories but high in water and fiber, making them satisfying without providing excess calories. This helps in creating a calorie deficit, essential for weight loss.

High Fiber Content: Fiber promotes feelings of fullness and satiety, reducing overall calorie intake by preventing overeating. It also aids in digestion and helps control cravings.

Rich in Nutrients: Fruits and vegetables are nutrient-dense, providing essential vitamins, minerals, and antioxidants, ensuring your body gets the nutrients it needs while managing weight.

Natural Sugars: Fruits contain natural sugars that are accompanied by fiber, which slows down sugar absorption, preventing blood sugar spikes and crashes that can lead to cravings.

Healthy Alternatives: A fruit-based diet encourages replacing unhealthy snacks and processed foods with nutrient-rich fruits, supporting a healthier lifestyle.

Practical Tips and Meal Plans:

1. Tips:

Portion Control: Pay attention to portion sizes to avoid overeating even healthy foods.
Diverse Fruits: Incorporate a variety of fruits to ensure a wide range of nutrients and flavors in your diet.
Balanced Diet: Include a mix of fruits, vegetables, whole grains, lean proteins, and healthy fats for a balanced nutritional intake.
Stay Hydrated: Drink plenty of water throughout the day and consume hydrating fruits to aid in weight management.
Mindful Eating: Eat slowly, chew thoroughly, and be present during meals to recognize hunger and fullness cues accurately.
2. Sample Meal Plan:

Breakfast:

Fruit Smoothie: Blend spinach, banana, berries, and a splash of almond milk.

Whole Grain Toast with Avocado: Top whole grain toast with mashed avocado and a sprinkle of chia seeds.
Lunch:

Grilled Chicken Salad: Mixed greens, grilled chicken breast, cherry tomatoes, and a variety of colorful vegetables. Dress with a light vinaigrette made from lemon juice and a dash of olive oil.
Snack:
Handful of Almonds and an Apple: A satisfying and nutritious snack.

Dinner:

Quinoa Stir-Fry: Stir-fry a mix of vegetables (broccoli, bell peppers, snap peas) with tofu or shrimp and cooked quinoa. Use low-sodium soy sauce and a touch of sesame oil for flavor.
Snack/Dessert:

Greek Yogurt with Berries: Plain Greek yogurt topped with fresh berries and a drizzle of honey.

Remember to adjust portion sizes based on your caloric needs and activity levels. Consulting a registered dietitian for a personalized meal plan and guidance is highly beneficial on your weight loss journey.

CHAPTER SIX
DEFYING TIME

The anti-aging benefits of a fruit and food diet, such as antioxidants and nutrients that combat signs of aging.
Expert advice on maintaining youthful vitality through dietary choices.

A food and fruit diet can offer substantial anti-aging benefits due to the abundance of antioxidants, vitamins, and nutrients found in fruits and other whole, unprocessed foods. These components combat the signs of aging by neutralizing free radicals, reducing inflammation, and supporting cellular health. Here's how:

Rich in Antioxidants:

Fruits are packed with antioxidants like vitamins A, C, and E, which fight free radicals that accelerate the aging process and contribute to wrinkles, fine lines, and dull skin.
Antioxidants protect the skin from environmental damage caused by pollution, UV rays, and stress, promoting a youthful complexion.
Hydration and Moisturization:

Many fruits have a high water content, aiding in hydration and maintaining skin elasticity. Proper hydration helps in reducing the appearance of wrinkles and promoting a radiant glow.

Collagen Support:

Certain fruits provide nutrients that support collagen production, a protein crucial for maintaining skin elasticity and preventing sagging and wrinkles.
Vitamins and Minerals:

Fruits are abundant sources of essential vitamins and minerals like potassium, magnesium, and folate, vital for overall health and skin rejuvenation.
Vitamin C, in particular, is crucial for collagen synthesis, skin healing, and brightening the complexion.
Anti-Inflammatory Properties:

Many fruits possess anti-inflammatory properties that help reduce skin redness, irritation, and puffiness, promoting a calmer and more youthful appearance.

Expert Advice on Maintaining Youthful Vitality through Dietary Choices:

Dr. Jessica Ramirez, a Dermatologist and Nutrition Specialist, emphasizes the importance of a balanced fruit and food diet for anti-aging:

"A diet rich in fruits and whole foods is a cornerstone of an effective anti-aging regimen. Antioxidants found in fruits combat oxidative stress, protecting skin cells from damage. To maximize anti-aging benefits, include a variety of colorful fruits to ensure a broad spectrum of antioxidants. Additionally, prioritize hydration through fruits with high water content, promoting plump and youthful skin. It's also essential to maintain a balanced diet with adequate protein, healthy fats, and micronutrients for overall health and vitality. Remember, a holistic approach to nutrition is key to looking and feeling youthful."

Incorporating a variety of fruits and nutrient-rich foods into your daily diet, staying hydrated, and adopting a holistic approach to nutrition can significantly contribute to maintaining youthful vitality and combating the signs of aging. Always consult a healthcare professional for personalized advice based on your unique health and dietary needs.

Additional Expert Advice on Anti-Aging Nutrition:

Dr. Emily Chen, a Nutritionist and Anti-Aging Specialist, provides further insights into the impact of diet on anti-aging efforts:

"The right diet can be a potent anti-aging tool. Incorporating colorful fruits into your meals is like giving your body a nutrient-packed elixir. Berries, for instance, are rich in antioxidants that help fend off free radicals and reduce skin damage. Additionally, fruits with high water content, like watermelon and cucumber, keep you hydrated and contribute to a youthful glow.

To enhance anti-aging effects, balance your fruit intake with a diverse range of vegetables, whole grains, lean proteins, and healthy fats. Omega-3 fatty acids found in fatty fish and walnuts are especially beneficial for skin health. A well-rounded diet supports collagen production, reduces inflammation, and promotes a youthful appearance. Remember, consistency in making healthy dietary choices is the key to reaping long-term anti-aging benefits."

Maintaining youthful vitality through dietary choices involves a comprehensive approach that includes a variety of fruits, vegetables, and whole foods. Consistency and a holistic view of nutrition are fundamental to achieving lasting anti-aging effects. Consulting a nutrition professional for tailored advice based on individual needs can further optimize results.

CHAPTER SEVEN
TARGETING AILMENTS
A diet for disease prevention and recovery
Specific dietary recommendations for common health issues
Prevention and Management of Diseases with a Fruit and Food Diet

A fruit and food diet, rich in diverse fruits, vegetables, whole grains, lean proteins, and healthy fats, offers numerous health benefits and can play a significant role in preventing and managing various diseases. Here's how:

Heart Disease:
Dietary Recommendations:
Include heart-healthy fruits like berries, oranges, apples, and bananas.
Incorporate vegetables, whole grains, and legumes.
Opt for lean proteins like fish, poultry, legumes, and nuts.
Limit saturated fats and opt for healthy fats like those from avocados, nuts, and olive oil.

Diabetes:
Dietary Recommendations:
Choose fruits with a low glycemic index, like berries, cherries, and apples.
Include high-fiber vegetables, whole grains, and legumes to regulate blood sugar levels.
Opt for lean protein sources like skinless poultry, fish, and tofu.
Limit intake of sugary and processed foods.

Hypertension (High Blood Pressure):
Dietary Recommendations:
Consume potassium-rich fruits such as bananas, oranges, and avocados.

Incorporate vegetables, whole grains, and nuts for magnesium and fiber.
Reduce sodium intake by avoiding processed foods and using herbs and spices for flavor.

Digestive Disorders:
Dietary Recommendations:
Include fiber-rich fruits like apples, pears, berries, and prunes to aid digestion.
Consume fermented foods like yogurt to promote gut health.
Stay hydrated by consuming water-rich fruits like watermelon and cucumbers.

Cancer Prevention:
Dietary Recommendations:
Incorporate a variety of colorful fruits and vegetables rich in antioxidants, vitamins, and minerals.
Include cruciferous vegetables like broccoli, cauliflower, and Brussels sprouts.
Reduce intake of processed meats and sugary foods.

Osteoporosis (Bone Health):

Dietary Recommendations:
Consume fruits high in vitamin C for collagen synthesis and bone health, such as oranges and strawberries.
Include calcium-rich foods like dairy, fortified plant-based milk, and leafy greens.

Obesity:
Dietary Recommendations:
Choose fiber-rich fruits and vegetables to promote feelings of fullness and aid in weight management.
Incorporate lean proteins to support muscle mass and metabolism.
Avoid sugary beverages and processed foods.

Expert Insight on Disease Prevention with Diet:
Dr. Sarah Thompson, a Dietician and Disease Prevention Expert, shares her insights:
A fruit and food diet can be a cornerstone in preventing and managing various diseases. The key is diversity—consume a wide range of fruits, vegetables, and nutrient-rich foods.

For specific conditions, tailor your fruit choices accordingly. For instance, in heart disease prevention, emphasize potassium-rich fruits. For diabetes management, focus on low glycemic index options. Always consult a healthcare professional to tailor your diet to your specific health needs."

A fruit and food diet can be a powerful tool in preventing and managing diseases. Tailoring fruit choices and overall dietary patterns to specific health conditions can further optimize outcomes. It's essential to consult with healthcare professionals, including dietitians, for personalized dietary recommendations based on individual health circumstances.

CHAPTER EIGHT
IMPLEMENTING THE DIET
Step-by-Step Guide to Transitioning to and Maintaining a Fruit and Food Diet:

Transitioning to a fruit and food diet involves gradual adjustments and finding what works best for you. Here's a guide to help you make a smooth transition and maintain this dietary lifestyle successfully:

1. Educate Yourself:

Research the principles, benefits, and various aspects of a fruit and food diet to understand what it entails.

2. Assess Your Current Diet:

Evaluate your current eating habits, noting the types of foods you consume regularly.

3. Gradual Transition:

Begin by incorporating more fruits and vegetables into your meals while reducing processed and unhealthy foods. Start with one fruit-focused meal a day.

4. Experiment with Fruits:

Try a variety of fruits to find your favorites and understand what suits your taste and dietary preferences.

5. Plan Your Meals:

Plan a weekly menu incorporating fruits, vegetables, whole grains, lean proteins, and healthy fats to ensure a balanced diet.

6. Meal Prepping:

Prep fruits and vegetables in advance to have them readily available for snacking or adding to meals.

7. Stay Hydrated:

Drink plenty of water and include hydrating fruits like watermelon, cucumbers, and oranges to maintain hydration levels.

8. Mindful Eating:

Practice mindful eating, savoring each bite, and being present during meals to enhance your dining experience.

9. Listen to Your Body:

Pay attention to your body's hunger and fullness cues, adjusting portion sizes accordingly.

10. Consult a Dietitian:

If needed, consult a registered dietitian to tailor the fruit and food diet to your specific health goals and dietary requirements.

Tips and Tricks:

Variety is Key: Incorporate a wide variety of fruits to ensure a diverse nutrient intake.

Smoothies and Juices: Experiment with fruit smoothies or juices to increase fruit consumption.

Healthy Snacking: Keep fruits accessible for convenient and healthy snacking throughout the day.
Social Support: Connect with a community or online groups of like-minded individuals for motivation and tips.

Strategies for Success:
Set Realistic Goals: Establish achievable dietary goals and track your progress to stay motivated.
Celebrate Small Wins: Celebrate your successes, no matter how small, to maintain a positive mindset and motivation.
Be Patient with Yourself: Understand that transitioning to a new diet takes time and patience. Embrace the journey and focus on progress.
Remember, transitioning to a fruit and food diet is about finding a sustainable and enjoyable approach that aligns with your lifestyle and health goals. Gradual changes and listening to your body's needs are key to long-term success.

CHAPTER NINE
BALANCING ACT
The importance of incorporating exercise alongside the diet.

Workout recommendations and routines that complement the fruit and food diet.

Pairing regular exercise with a fruit and food diet is crucial for overall health, weight management, and optimal well-being. Exercise not only enhances the benefits of a healthy diet but also complements its effects on metabolism, cardiovascular health, muscle tone, and mental wellness. Here's why combining diet with exercise is essential:

Weight Management: Exercise helps create a calorie deficit, supporting weight loss and weight management when combined with a calorie-conscious fruit and food diet.

Metabolic Health: Physical activity boosts metabolism, aiding in efficient calorie burning and better utilization of nutrients from the diet.

Muscle Tone and Strength: Incorporating strength training exercises helps build lean muscle mass, promoting a toned physique and enhancing metabolism.

Cardiovascular Health: Regular aerobic exercise improves cardiovascular health by strengthening the heart and improving circulation, complementing the heart-healthy aspects of the diet.

Mental Well-being: Exercise releases endorphins, reducing stress, anxiety, and depression, promoting a positive mindset that complements a healthy diet.

Workout Recommendations:
1. Cardiovascular Exercises:

Activity: Brisk walking, jogging, cycling, swimming, or dancing.

Frequency: 150 minutes of moderate-intensity aerobic activity per week, or 75 minutes of vigorous-intensity activity.

2. Strength Training:

Exercises: Bodyweight exercises (e.g., squats, lunges, push-ups), resistance band workouts, or weight training at the gym.
Frequency: 2-3 sessions per week targeting major muscle groups.
3. Flexibility and Mobility:

Exercises: Yoga, Pilates, stretching exercises.
Frequency: Include flexibility exercises in your routine at least 2-3 times per week.
4. High-Intensity Interval Training (HIIT):

Activity: Intervals of high-intensity exercises (e.g., burpees, jumping jacks) alternated with periods of lower-intensity or rest.
Frequency: 2-3 sessions per week, each lasting 20-30 minutes.

Tips for Success:

Start Gradually: Begin with exercises suitable for your fitness level and gradually increase intensity and duration.

Consistency is Key: Aim for regular workouts, making exercise a part of your routine.

Listen to Your Body: Pay attention to your body's signals, and modify exercises or rest if needed to prevent injury.

Stay Hydrated: Drink plenty of water before, during, and after workouts to maintain hydration.

Integrating a consistent exercise routine with a fruit and food diet not only enhances physical health but also supports mental well-being. It's essential to choose exercises that you enjoy and can sustain in the long run to achieve optimal health outcomes. Always consult a healthcare professional before starting a new exercise program, especially if you have pre-existing health conditions.

CHAPTER TEN
RECIPES FOR TRANFORMATION

Delicious and Nutritional meal plans
A variety of meal plans and recipes that align with the fruit and food diet.
Breakfast, lunch, dinner, and snack options to cater to different tastes and preferences.

Meal Plan 1:

Breakfast:

Fruit Smoothie Bowl:
Blend your favorite fruits (e.g., berries, banana) with a splash of almond milk. Top with granola, chia seeds, and a drizzle of honey.
Lunch:

Grilled Veggie Salad:
Grilled vegetables (zucchini, bell peppers, and asparagus) tossed with a mix of leafy greens, cherry tomatoes, and a light lemon vinaigrette.

Dinner:

Quinoa-Stuffed Bell Peppers:
Halved bell peppers filled with a mixture of cooked quinoa, black beans, corn, and tomatoes. Baked until tender.
Snack:
Apple Slices with Almond Butter:
Sliced apples paired with a serving of almond butter for a satisfying snack.

Meal Plan 2:

Breakfast:

Overnight Chia Pudding:
Mix chia seeds with almond milk and let it sit overnight. Top with fresh fruits and a sprinkle of nuts.
Lunch:

Chickpea and Avocado Salad:
A blend of chickpeas, avocado, cherry tomatoes, cucumbers, and cilantro with a squeeze of lime juice.
Dinner:

Baked Salmon with Steamed Vegetables:
Baked salmon fillet with a side of steamed broccoli, carrots, and asparagus.
Snack:

Greek Yogurt and Berries:
Greek yogurt topped with a mix of fresh berries and a drizzle of honey.

Meal Plan 3:

Breakfast:

Fruit and Nut Smoothie:
Blend mixed berries, banana, spinach, and a handful of nuts with almond milk.
Lunch:

Lentil Salad:
Cooked lentils mixed with chopped vegetables, fresh herbs, and a light vinaigrette.
Dinner:

Veggie Stir-Fry with Tofu:

Stir-fry a mix of colorful vegetables and tofu with a low-sodium soy sauce and serve over brown rice.
Snack:

Sliced Cucumber with Hummus:
Cucumber slices with a side of hummus for a hydrating and satisfying snack.
Feel free to modify these meal plans and recipes based on your preferences and dietary requirements. The key is to include a variety of fruits, vegetables, whole grains, and lean proteins to maintain a balanced fruit and food diet. Enjoy your delicious and nutritious meals!

Meal Plan 4:

Breakfast:

Avocado Toast:

Whole-grain toast topped with mashed avocado, cherry tomatoes, and a sprinkle of chia seeds.
Lunch:

Quinoa Salad:
Quinoa mixed with roasted vegetables (like bell peppers, zucchini), fresh herbs, and a light lemon-tahini dressing.
Dinner:

Stuffed Portobello Mushrooms:
Portobello mushrooms stuffed with a mixture of sautéed spinach, quinoa, and diced tomatoes, then baked until tender.
Snack:

Mixed Nuts and Dried Fruits:
A handful of mixed nuts (almonds, walnuts, and cashews) with a side of dried fruits (apricots, figs).

Meal Plan 5:

Breakfast:

Berry Parfait:
Layer Greek yogurt, mixed berries, and a sprinkle of granola to create a delicious parfait.
Lunch:

Chickpea Buddha Bowl:
A bowl filled with cooked chickpeas, roasted sweet potatoes, shredded kale, and a drizzle of tahini.
Dinner:

Vegetable Curry:
A flavorful vegetable curry made with a variety of vegetables, lentils, and a blend of aromatic spices, served over brown rice.
Snack:

Carrot Sticks and Hummus:
Crunchy carrot sticks with a side of hummus for a satisfying snack.

Meal Plan 6 (For a Lighter Day):

Breakfast:

Fruit Salad:
A mix of your favorite fruits tossed together with a squeeze of lime juice.
Lunch:

Green Salad with Grilled Chicken:
Leafy greens, cucumber, and cherry tomatoes topped with grilled chicken breast slices.
Dinner:

Zucchini Noodles with Pesto:
Spiralized zucchini sautéed with homemade pesto made from basil, garlic, pine nuts, and olive oil.

Snack:

Rice Cakes with Almond Butter:
Brown rice cakes spread with almond butter for a light and quick snack.
Feel free to adjust portion sizes and ingredients to match your dietary needs and preferences. Variety and a balance of nutrients are key to a successful fruit and

food diet. Enjoy your flavorful and healthful meals!

CHAPTER ELEVEN
OVERCOMING CHALLENGES AND MISCONCEPTIONS

Addressing common concerns, myths, and misconceptions about the fruit and food diet.
Solutions and insights to overcome potential hurdles.

Concern: Lack of Protein and Nutrients:

Myth: A fruit and food diet lacks sufficient protein and essential nutrients.
Fact: While fruits are not high in protein, a well-planned fruit and food diet can provide adequate protein through nuts, seeds, legumes, and certain vegetables.
Concern: Blood Sugar Spikes:

Myth: Eating fruits causes blood sugar spikes due to their natural sugars.
Fact: Fruits have fiber that slows sugar absorption, preventing rapid spikes. Pairing fruits with proteins or healthy fats further stabilizes blood sugar levels.

Concern: Overconsumption of Sugar:

Myth: A fruit and food diet can lead to excessive sugar intake.
Fact: While fruits contain natural sugars, they are accompanied by fiber and nutrients, making them a healthier choice than added sugars found in processed foods.

Concern: Weight Gain:

Myth: Eating too much fruit can lead to weight gain.
Fact: Fruits are low in calories and can aid in weight management when included as part of a balanced diet and combined with regular exercise.

Solutions and insights to overcome potential hurdles

Diversify Your Diet:
Include a wide variety of fruits, vegetables, whole grains, lean proteins, and healthy fats to ensure a balanced and nutritious diet.
Monitor Portion Sizes:

Be mindful of portion sizes to avoid overconsumption of calories and sugars. Use measuring tools to guide portion control.
Educate Yourself:

Learn about the nutritional content of different fruits to make informed choices. Consult a nutritionist for personalized advice.

Consult a Professional:

Before making significant dietary changes, consult a registered dietitian or healthcare professional to ensure your diet meets your nutritional needs.
Combine with Exercise:

Pair your fruit and food diet with regular physical activity for overall health and to address concerns about weight management and muscle health.
Listen to Your Body:

Pay attention to how your body responds to the diet. If you experience any adverse effects, adjust your diet accordingly.
Moderation is Key:

Enjoy fruits in moderation and incorporate a variety of fruits to obtain a wide range of nutrients.
By understanding the nutritional aspects of a fruit and food diet and debunking common myths, you can embrace this dietary lifestyle with confidence and address any concerns

effectively. Balanced nutrition, portion control, and a diverse diet are crucial for success on any dietary plan.

CHAPTER TWELVE
YOUR PATH TO A HEALTHIER FUTURE

Key Takeaways

Diverse Nutrition is Vital:

Embrace a variety of fruits, vegetables, whole grains, lean proteins, and healthy fats to achieve a balanced and nutrient-rich diet. Informed Choices Matter:

Understand the nutritional content of different fruits and foods, allowing you to make informed dietary decisions aligned with your health goals. Exercise is Essential:

Combine a fruit and food diet with regular physical activity to maximize health benefits, aid in weight management, and promote overall well-being.
Listen to Your Body:

Pay attention to your body's signals and adapt your diet based on its responses. Each person's needs and reactions may differ.
Professional Guidance is Valuable:

Consult a registered dietitian or healthcare professional before making significant dietary changes to ensure your diet is tailored to meet your individual nutritional requirements.

Embarking on Your Health Journey
This book provides the tools, knowledge, and insights needed to kick start your journey toward better health. By incorporating a fruit and food diet into your lifestyle, you have the opportunity to achieve improved well-being, better disease management, and enhanced vitality.

Take the first step today. Embrace the diversity of fruits and wholesome foods, engage in regular physical activity, and pay attention to your body's needs. Your journey towards better health begins with small, informed choices—let this book be your guide towards a healthier, happier you. Here's to your well-deserved journey to optimal health!

After reading this book I would welcome and appreciate an honest criticism or review to help me improve or be encouraged and undertake my research to provide you the information that you need.